Descent into Dementia: Who Am I and where are We Now?

Descent into Dementia: Who Am I and where are We Now?

Karen J. Chism

Large Print Edition

Heartspeak Publications Incorporated
heartspeakpublications@gmail.com

DESCENT INTO DEMENTIA:
WHO AM I AND WHERE ARE WE NOW?

~*~

Published by Heartspeak Publications Incorporated, Michigan, USA

heartspeakpublications@gmail.com
chism.karenj@gmail.com

Unless otherwise noted, any references to: The Holy Bible, The Bible, or God's Word, refer to direct quotes or the author's paraphrasing of scripture from THE HOLY BIBLE, *KING JAMES VERSION.*

Acknowledgements

Once again—as with all my writings, I express my deep appreciation for my Editor in Chief — K. Compton. She is a fine woman and I don't mind saying so—it isn't my doing, so it is not my pride speaking. Without her expertise in the new technology, correcting my many blunders, I would not live long enough to have my work—*print ready*!

Love ya

I thank my God, through my Lord and Savior Jesus Christ, for the inspiration and the strength to express myself in rhymes.
My prayer, desire, and mission—may all I write bring honor and glory to Him.

Preface

Why a book of poems devoted entirely to narrating the day-to-day devastation and challenges that accompany Dementia?

My health drastically limits my ability to vocalize; that coupled with Jim's decreasing cognitive functions; evolved quite naturally into my penchant for writing and rhyming. Additionally, my surprise realization that, even with all the resources of this great nation—some professionals are woefully ignorant regarding some mental illnesses.

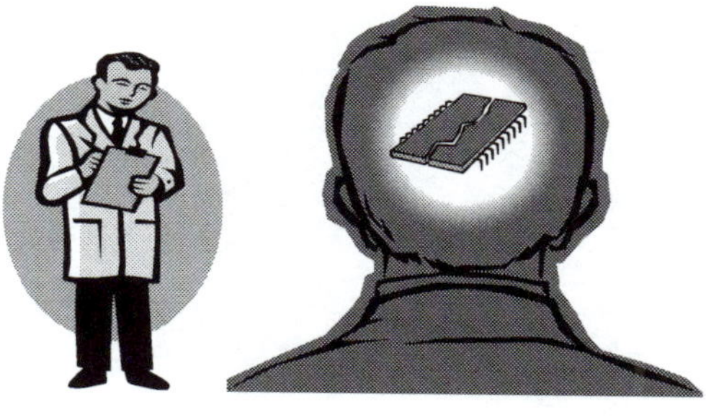

Dementia with Lewy Bodies is a complex blend of: Alzheimer's memory loss and confusion; the slow stiffness of Parkinson's; and, the paranoia and hallucinations of Schizophrenia.

Perhaps, through exposing our painful personal experiences; others may not only feel some kinship but derive a measure of hope while trudging through this life altering disease.

I appreciated the book by Kirk Hall, "Window of Opportunity."[3] It was very helpful to me, and I highly recommend it—especially for someone new to the struggle—with the alarming changes taking place in their life. Mr. Hall's experiences and symptoms were much like my Jim's in the earlier days of the disease.

Table of Contents

Wannabe Doctors

I have been told, "Jim can't have Alzheimer's because—
My grandmother has it and Jim doesn't act like *she* does"

One man declared—No one who can recite John 3:16 perfectly—
Could possibly have Dementia, that's for certainty

Another has determined—Jim remembers the words of a song—
They sang together as children, therefore; I'm lying and wrong

With all the hours these wannabe doctors spend on the internet
Diagnosing to suit their own agenda hasn't improved their intellect

Wannabe doctors cause a myriad of trouble
Crushing whole families into a heap of rubble!

~*~

All Alone

The tears are never far from my eyes
Accompanying my silent petitions and cries

God—though I know You are with me
I crave more conversation with Thee

I have no one in this world by my side
To hold my hand on this painful ride

My breath comes in sobs obstructing my speech
Praying; my pain to God's throne it would reach

"Till death do us part," was our vow long ago
Never suspecting together we'd face all this woe

His frail body I care for best as I can; though I'm weak
Strength to carry on comes only from The Lord I seek

Gasping for air to keep life in this body each hour
Struggling to help with our daily shower

Heartbreaking sadness overwhelms me today
Other people's happiness accentuates our decay

Not much joy in our world today can I find
Any happiness is in memories of the mind

Although I have only pain here and now
Bittersweet memories is all circumstances will allow

My throat feels crushed holding back my tears
Probably, nobody but You Lord, knows my fears

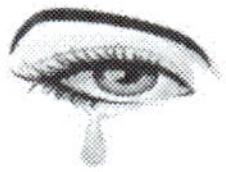

Through sickness and health—
The hunger and the wealth

These were the promises we made
We would face them together; unafraid

But this—you left me all alone
To face the pain and unknown

Hearts can break from loneliness I do believe
The load is so heavy; without a reprieve

My tears at the ready; my vision to cloud
With Dementia there is no sharing allowed

Karen J. Chism 12/25/2014—Christmas morning

Descent into Dementia

Alzheimer's and Dementia has a head start long before the diagnosis
Sometimes it manifests as an irritating inability to focus

It may appear that a loved one is not giving you their attention
A need to repeat, because their difficulty with retention

Doors are left open and water still flowing
Little things really; without his knowing

More absent minded, forgetting daily routine
Avoidance—is the preferred smoke screen

Hallucinations we excused as sleepwalking
That act is accepted and far less shocking

The visual disturbances while he is awake
Those, soon become hard for any to mistake

The pressure the afflicted experiences; wanting to hide
Might result in a dangerous psychotic slide

This is our story—told in my preferred writing
style
A compilation of daily events; praying my effort
will be considered worthwhile

Dementia is a cruel disease, affecting the family
as well as the afflicted
The closer the relationship, the greater the hurt;
no one could have predicted

As the victim of the illness, travels more
frequently in a world of their own
The spouse must painfully, watch their love one
leaving; grieving and alone

It is true his body resides in our home as usual
But I can't share the trip of his mind; the
delusional

He talks to me of things that are not happening
or real
The disease robbed his discernment; I watched it
steal

I struggle with an appropriate response to his
imaginary observations
Not wanting to anger or belittle his declarations

As I watch my handsome man's body, through my unshed tears
Make physical changes far greater than just years

As he complains of the inability to describe what is going on in his head
I helplessly observe his skeletal configuration changes—with dread

However, the heartbreak I can't adequately express
With each new day and night the illness does progress

This man—that was so intellectual in the past
The changes magnifying a *gigantic contrast*

He is frightened and so unsure of himself, not able to even trust what he sees
Simple objects like a chair, morph in his gaze to various degrees

It must be such a nightmare for him to not even recognize his own shirt
Some things, sometimes, are familiar to him but he is less and less alert

I've tried every form of entertainment to manage the depression
Yet, even a child's game is out of the question

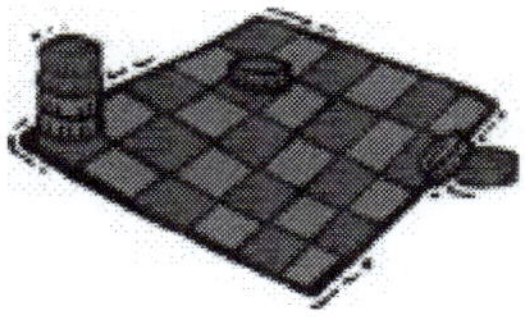

Thankfully he still knows me and calls me by name
I have to face the possibility it might not remain the same

But sometimes he will imagine I am just across the room
And when I don't answer, then his anger will resume

We moved from our familiar home of 20 years
Maybe that has contributed to some of his fears

But—as I think back—that's probably not the case
Oft times, he didn't know where he was, at the old place

So far he recognizes family members when he sees them all right
His problem is that he sees people when nobody is here all day and night

He will speak to them, but gets upset because the *vase of flowers* doesn't answer his talk
He'll get angry and right over to the *object* he will walk

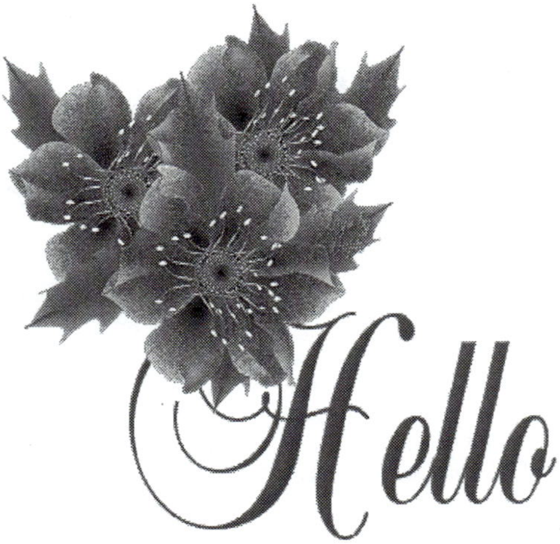

A bit ago, he was being a good host and offered a friend from the past
A bottle of water and tried to hand it to him as he asked

Of course there was nobody but the two of us in the room
I silently watched him turn away, his face full of gloom

It is so sad, but the doctor said these aberrations are very real to him
How painful it is to see this happen to my Jim

So much needs to be discovered regarding the death of our body's cells
We know the effect of the destruction on the organs as well

Dementia plays no favorites among rich, poor, or educated
Male, female, or famous and celebrated

There is nothing quite like it; I judge it is the worst
Your body lives long after your mind gave up first

It is awful to watch my loved one realize he is
losing his mind and cannot change
This stage I can only believe is worse than when
everything will be strange

When the mind *does* go completely he won't
know what he doesn't know
I have seen examples of persons in that state and
they aren't as miserable; they go with the flow

My love often says to me, "Come on, let's go
home"
I try to reassure him we *ARE* home—through the
house he does roam

There are just short periods these days where he
can be brought into reality
These indeed are treasured moments of
normalcy

I witness him traveling from here to God only
knows where
In a matter of seconds; so, I need always be
aware

He will think that he sees me sitting at my desk in the den
To the family room he will come get me to go with him and then

He will be upset because I didn't talk to him before
Insisting that all I did was ignore

I try to explain that I can't be two places at once *and was not there*
I can't convince him even though he just pokes at the air

Each day brings more torment for him in his confused mind
It surely is in an *evil prison* of sorts he's confined

He told me today that he has lost his identity
Sadly right along with it goes his dignity

He said he is afraid to be around people if he will have to talk
Never knowing if the person is even there—or if they'll mock

These days Dementia is more recognized and empathy it brings
Seems as though everyone knows or has known somebody with a similar thing

The biggest problem, as I see it and fear
He's becoming more agitated and aggression does appear

This is not a normal state for him to be in
He has always faced life with a positive spin

Being a doctor himself, he is definitely aware of the hopeless prognosis
He is cognizant enough to observe his own psychosis

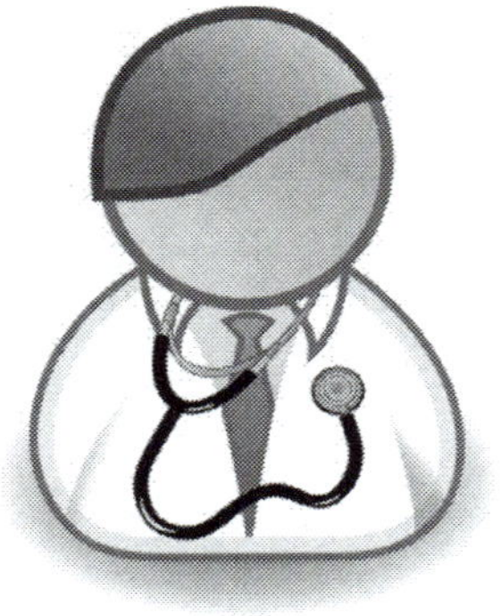

He has spent his adult life dealing with other people's pain
Sad when a healer can't help himself; try as he might it's all in vain

It is a rare thing these days to see a smile on his face
The deep frown lines on his brow have the prominent place

His huge grin was his very best feature, though his sense of humor's not far behind
He loved to tease the grandkids, but was never unkind

As I look over the verses I have written above
I speak a lot in the past tense, but . . . much is vanished of my love

He acts out what he describes as his dreams
This is a frightening aspect, if they have dangerous themes

I can only trust and pray that my Lord
Knows what's going on and has not ignored

The **Lord's Will** I accept; what will be done regardless
Up until now my love's actions though upsetting are harmless

Harmless in that he has not caused any physical, obvious pain
But the heart and mind ache isn't always visible, that we sustain

We are *both* prisoners as his paranoid state evolves
Just praying soon that research; the illness will resolve

This cruel disease has taken a turn for the worst the past couple of weeks
I know I was told by a wise physician it would have valleys and peaks

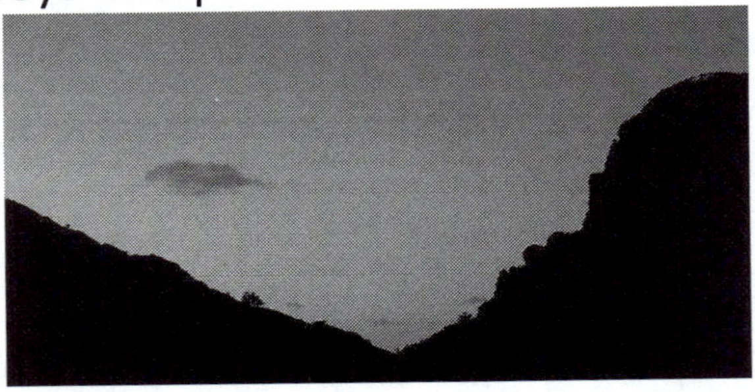

But the valleys are lower and peaks not so high
It is so hard to observe this happening to my guy

He doesn't know where he is, most of the hours night or day
I dare not be out of his sight or the paranoia has its way

I search the internet for answers but there is
none
**I don't even know what to pray for; except His
Will be done**

I know my love is suffering so; he can't even
express the agony of his dreams
He can't begin to sort out reality or hallucinations
it seems

It is getting harder for him to take all the
confusion in stride
Having more angry outbursts, as his hope is
denied

Today he can't find his way in the house without
my leading by the hand
Heartbreaking that he can't follow the simplest
command

Come, let's eat in the kitchen and come to the
table
He can't do that on his own, no he is not able

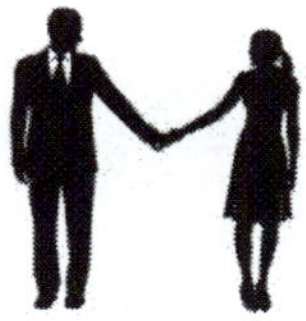

He is not sleeping at night and it is taking its toll on me
I need one eye on him so where he goes I can see

This getting old business is not for wimps, I tell you
There are some that live to the end with good health it is true

But one never knows if they'll be among the many or the few
There are all kinds of illness that one may get, but Dementia . . . whew!

I personally know what a blow it is to be told you have the "Big C"
However, I think it is even more painful to have the "Big D"

After a week of not sleeping, bringing both my love and me down
Went to the neurologist got the mildest medicine that is found

My love slept for 13 hours last night
Woke up this morning, seemed more bright

I know it is temporary, but I take the good with the bad
Good days are rare now, and that's is *just* so sad

A simple request to bring attention to an object
The direction I point in, he can't locate or detect

I can explain the article he wants is on the table
Maybe five repetitions before finding he is able

One purpose in documenting all the phases and changes
As I witness 24/7, is to illuminate the ranges

For a ten minute visit with a physician
Who performs a standard test for cognition

I do believe I have a suggestion to improve
The patient and caregiver it would behoove

Giving the caregiver a questionnaire to fill
May help the doctor choose the correct pill

The neurologist admitted, "It is a joint experiment"
No one can predict individual development

A bit of a fright today, while I was out of the room
My love, he talked to me; my not answering, he fumed

He started the van but could not operate the gears
Dangerous situation ensued; called 911 with my fears

They talked him into giving me the keys
I anticipate there may be more times like these

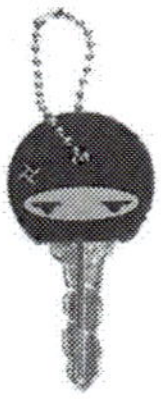

The policeman told my husband a small fib that day
Saying he didn't have a valid driver's license; to not drive away

Today my love announced in a matter of fact way
"I can't drive any more . . . at all, they say"

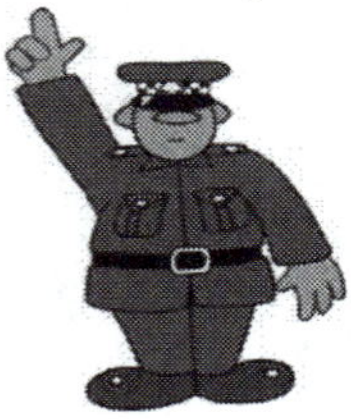

I was thankful he believed the officer without a fight
I've tried; couldn't accomplish this with all my might

I pray I will be able to manage these horrible dangers
I don't want my love to have to live among strangers

No doubt there will come a time, he won't know me
God alone knows; He holds the progression time-table, you see

Paranoia is becoming a really big deal
Hallucinations; causing problems unreal

Now, he has repeated visions of men in my bed
Breaking his heart and mine into shreds!

I have always slept with extra pillows between my knees
Now they morph into men having sex; *oh please!*

Several times a day now he will matter-of-factly ask me
"Say, what is that guy's name; the one that sleeps here with thee?"

How can he have a recurring hallucination so vivid, yet untrue?
I don't understand it and none of the physicians have a clue!

Neither one of us were ever unfaithful in our married life
We have been very satisfied together living without strife

He thinks I have men in my bed every night; but can't remember their name
How troubling it must be for him; what a terrible shame

Of all the hallucinations he relates in great detail
imagining other men is the most distressing travail

He asks me, "What are we going to do about it?"
Saying, "I can't take it, are we going to split?"

How heartbreaking is that, to think your wife in the next bed
Has other men with her and to her they aren't wed

He often inquires as to my boyfriend's name
I know he can't help it, but what a shame!

I take him on a tour of the bed every night, to feel the pillows are not a man
But he insists they come in the middle of the night; assuring me—"They can"

The fireplace is just one object he has talks with every day
Scary, sometimes when they answer him; in an evil way

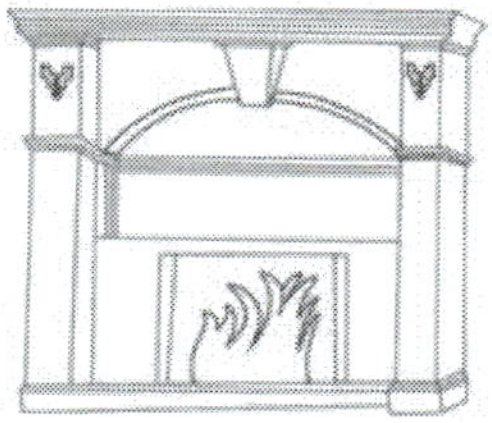

My love asked me, "Do you have to work today?"
I answered, "No, I'm home all day," that seemed okay

"What are those other people going to be doing?"
Of course, I don't see them or what he is viewing

"Nobody here but the two of us," I say
He snickers at me in a disgusted way

"Where are those other people going to sleep tonight?"
I walk him through all the rooms to show that it is all right

He will close the bedroom door for privacy from other folks
He'd been doing this for years; I didn't catch what it evokes

Some symptoms materialized subtlety over time
Others as drastic as an exploding land mine

It has been ignorantly exclaimed, by many causing great pain
How could he have Dementia yet, correctly diagnose and explain?

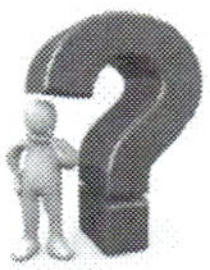

Different parts of the brain are responsible for certain actions
One may remember how to treat an illness
but, not the answer to a simple 3rd grade fraction

Scientists and physicians have many theories to speak
Answers still escape them so, continually they seek

Meanwhile families try to hold it together and cope
For all the experts; *none* give us any hope

My love now has trouble when I am talking; looking directly in my eyes
It requires concentration and causes a headache he does advise

He explains the same thing happens when trying to read a book
After a few minutes; away he must look

The majority of the time he stares off into space
Therefore his mind wonders and the hallucinations take place

I observe he's much like a child that has a problem paying attention
It is not a matter of memory but rather concentration

I did some research for Lewy bodies on the internet today
Some believe there's a connection with ADHD they say

I do see the similarities and tend to agree
By observing 24/7; though I've no formal degree

His symptoms *differ* from Alzheimer's in presentation
Memory loss not the big thing but confusion and aberration

His memory can't be trusted, the hallucinations are so real
That is the major problem with his type of Dementia; security it doth steal

One example; he might inquire of me
"Where will I sleep tonight, a place I don't see?"

Walking back and forth out in the hall
Unsure how to get ready for bed; he can't recall

Forgetting to swallow; results in drooling
Gives the impression; no manners or schooling

That is not the case; rather normal function
Body movements; reflexes lost conjunction

Once Dementia gets a strong hold
Body functions are usually uncontrolled

End stages of Dementia bring an inability to eat
Swallowing eventually becomes a major feat

Changing his shoes from the black pair to the tan
A major accomplishment, after six tries he can

Concentration poses a daily war with confusion
Too often the victor is an optical illusion

No wonder paranoia is a part of the disease
Never certain if it is real or not; what he sees

My poor Jim had a superior IQ before dementia took it away
Sometimes we spell for our sweet Yorkie who learns more words every day

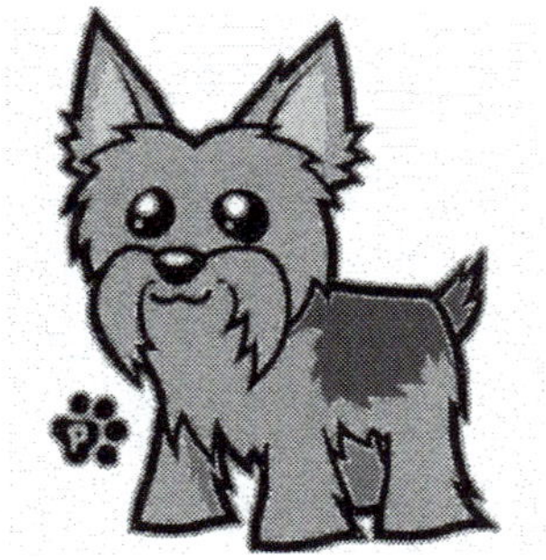

Now when I ask my Jim to go for a w-a-l-k
He looks at me blankly not knowing what I spell or say

To vocalize is frustrating and confusing to replay
I need to take his hand most times and lead the way

Yet his ***understanding changes*** every hour
What it may be in 15 minutes, he has no power

He spends hour after hour, eyes closed to the world around him
Opportunity to draw him into reality is slim

He says even watching a ball game hurts his head
Things he used to enjoy, he now dreads

It is so painful for me to see him this way
I called him "silver tongue," he could debate all day

My love proclaimed today, "I have the strangest feeling—
That I'm detached from my mind," heartbreaking but revealing

Glen Campbell wrote a song for his wife Kim
"I'm Not Goanna Miss You,"[1] so brave of him

I barely managed to listen to the song's end
Jim won't miss me; but my grief will transcend

We are at a new low; although for now under control
Jim can't shower himself; but allowing help—our goal

Always a very private man it was very hard
To allow others in his space; formerly barred

My own illness prevents performing certain tasks
Thankfully we can hire helpers, to do whatever he asks

It is more difficult to go out to a restaurant to eat
Hallucinations cause anxiety not the anticipated treat

His speech is getting harder to understand every day
He knows what he is thinking and trying to say

Yet when asked to repeat; he will quickly forget
Can't ask too many times for then he gets upset

He will go through his wallet looking carefully at each card
Saying he needs to be sure when the cops ask it won't be too hard

Though he has a hundred dollar bill in his wallet and a credit card too
A few bucks in his pocket over and over he withdrew

He knows money is important of this he is sure
Not knowing what to do with it; just makes him feel insecure

It is increasingly difficult to look at the man I love
Over three years now; only reminiscent of

In photos he looked like he knew what was relevant
In person now the confused look is permanent

It is hard to explain other than a portion of life is gone
Some cells in his brain are indeed dead; visually withdrawn

I keep looking and hoping for some sign the old Jim will be here
It is hard to accept with the myriad of cells; the big changes that appear

Jim explained today the problem with conversation
The inability for continuity breeds agitation

He starts with a thought to share with me
Forgetting in the middle of the sentence you see

I try to help him out, by gently asking "What did you say?"
I think that frustrates him more in some way

Sometimes I think it is better to just change the subject
Lets him off the hook—frustration it does deflect

It does make me feel like I am not paying attention
But if he feels snubbed—I know he lacks retention

With so much progress in science you would think they could find
A lot more about brain cells and replace the faulty parts of the mind

Some will explain a faulty function as forgetting
But I see it as a lack of continuity—upsetting

A simple example we all have experienced many times
Going into a room and forgetting what we came for sometimes

When this is the case with most of his moves
It's no wonder paranoia ensues

It seems there will always be those that only look for a blame
Not enough attention paid to quality of life—it's a shame

I have noticed this week a progression in the disease
It is more difficult to get his attention; lost by degrees

I can call him to dinner at least six times and look right at him
Most times I need to touch or guide; pulling by a limb

Conversation is limited to a couple of words to speak
The chance for a whole sentence of thought now is bleak

He will stop in the middle of a thought attempting to communicate
Left with only a blank canvas to hallucinate

Those critical of his lack of attention
Don't have a clue as to his limited retention

My love is here in my house, yet he is gone from the room
A myriad of misconceptions less familiar persons presume

Shallow people never having experienced the horror and pain
Do nothing to help; just know how to complain

Cruel to heap pressure to change back to the past
The lack of compassion for the illness; I'm aghast!

Looking for fixes and someone to blame
Trashing relationships; everyone is fair game

There is a stranger living in my house less familiar each day
An occasional shadow exposes a likeness replay

The smile that *escapes* over the constant frown
Lets me know my Jim is still in there; still around

There is this tiny spark that is still connected
Trying my best for him to feel protected

The isolation that results without a human connection
True intimacy is impossible without the recollection

Sometimes I feel I have lost Jim a long time ago
Unable to express spontaneously, ya know

Forced into the position of caregiver instead of wife
Overshadows intimate recognition—changes our life

True love necessitates compassion and care
Dementia robbed us of the closeness we did formerly share

Marital sex for us includes a blending of the mind
Not just for fun; or the sensuous kind

When the connection is broken between body and mind
As it is with Dementia; a *different* relationship is assigned

We will deal with it all one day at a time
I'll record the puzzles as they unfurl; in rhyme

We had visitors over for dinner today
A greeting was ignored; not even a "Hey"

I perceive hallucinations are so many for Jim
He has learned to ignore most since he can't win

When a vision is reality he doesn't recognize it
A few minutes later he doesn't remember a bit

Thankful for the caregivers and helpers each day
Allowing us to remain in our home; making a way

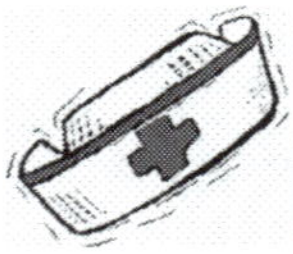
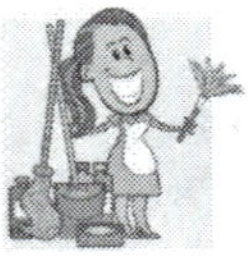
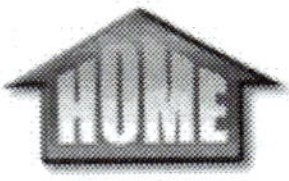

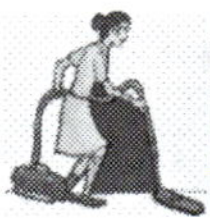
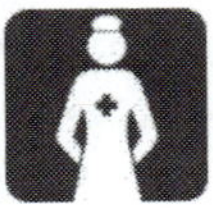

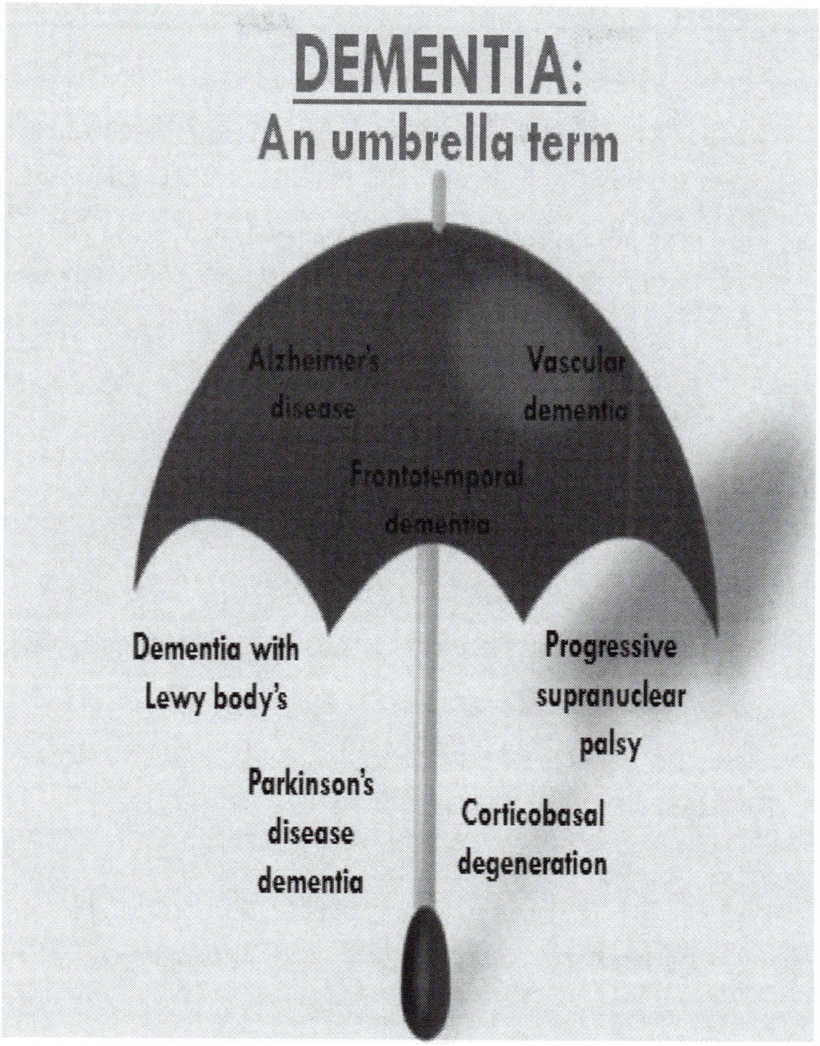

Accepting the duality of being absent yet present
the *long bumpy road of Descent into Dementia*

I Have No Idea What I Know

[Kris, Ashley, and I were talking about cheese. Kris asked what "Head Cheese" is. Ashley explained and then I asked Jim, "Do you know about Head Cheese?" Jim said, with an adorable *smirk,* **"I have no idea what I know."** *2/26/2015*]

Jim *might* say:

I don't know—what I know; why do you ask?
The recalling has become too great a task

If I have the answer, part is obscured
Can't tell you till, damn Dementia is cured!

But we can still laugh at shortcomings today
Sense of humor God gave me is still okay

On occasion I'll share a peak of my former wisdom with you
Then you can declare with pride—Jim knew!

Hanging by a Thread

Sometimes I feel like I'm hanging on by a thread; but that is wrong
If only by a thin thread; I would have long been gone

To give any credit to that proverbial thread isn't fair
For really, that kind of thinking is an evil snare

I *do know* where the thanks should be placed
I pray I won't ever forget; no matter what I face

This morning at my rehab session, a therapist named Diane
Explained to me, the Monarch butterflies' game plan

She brought to work, a container of four butterflies ready to hatch
I was amazed as they broke through the covering, and by a **silk thread** they were attached

I was honored to let one of the four fly free
A truly amazing sight to see

She explained it was a female, and showed me how to tell
Her soft gentle narration put me in a spell

The delicate creature needed to fly from Michigan to Mexico
How it could ever manage that, only God can know

I wondered about the thread I feel like I'm hanging from
I envisioned my flight—further then Mexico—when The Lord Jesus says, "Come"

—And some say, "There is no God"
The strength of that thread; I'm awed!

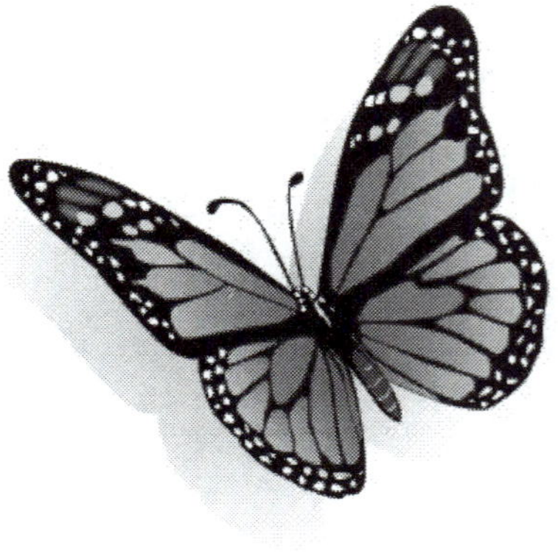

Karen J. Chism 8/26/2014

The Big "C" and "D"

Both my love and I have serious afflictions
These necessitate uncommon restrictions

For he is unable to comprehend—let alone assist
But with God's Grace we are able to coexist

Because he was a physician and more educated then me
The loss of his cognitive ability is terrifying, you see

I trusted and looked to him for medical advice
Now he cannot even recall I have cancer; to be precise

I have been battling four different cancers, for 18 years now
I could never have survived without The Lord—no how

When my first tumor was discovered in my breast
My love didn't have to think twice; sent me for a fast and a rest

I went out of state for a 45 day water fast
My Jim recommended; I didn't question or ask

My love made the long drive, two times a week
None of my roommates had visitors; I was unique

He surprised me and balanced our books to the penny
Ten years later I went back again; mistakes were aplenty

This time, I had to come home after just 14 days
By then his memory left the books in a maze

He couldn't find his way to visit and got lost
I couldn't leave him to drive alone at any cost

After my mastectomy we went vegan for five long years
Then I got a large tumor; had to remove the whole lung; more tears

Jim was still pretty sharp at that time and very attentive
Would get me anything I thought I might eat for an incentive

That surgery was pretty rough; it almost "got me"
But The Lord was with us, surely you'd agree

Tumor number three came about five years later
Now the other lung; taking a lobe left a crater

By this time my love was having greater problems with his mind
Visiting me in the hospital, the exit he couldn't find

Two months after my new surgery, Jim had a breakdown
He was hospitalized almost four months; I was still run-down

One year later; in my only lung—tumor number four
The surgeon couldn't cut out any more

Jim's Dementia gets worse every day
My prognosis is dire but God has His way

We are blessed that we have been able to find
Home helpers and caregivers—so very kind

The unusual predicament in our situation
Received harm—not help from his blood relation

As Jim becomes increasingly more dependent
Unfortunately I too become interdependent

He can't shower or dress himself at this time
Or most nights how to get into bed he can't find

Can't figure out how to pull up the covers
Simple things are problematic, we discover

The *physical requirements* of day-to-day living take a toll
As I grow weaker and his mind has a bigger hole

If people's memories bring satisfaction
Their absence—must have a greater anxiety reaction

Dementia is a "twofer" the spouse knows for sure
For the life changing challenges—there is no instruction brochure

Unable to dress or undress himself these days
Requires strength from another in a myriad ways

He is so sweet; he does try by himself to do
Must be horribly frustrating; can't put on his shoe

He'll put his arms in his pant legs and it doesn't work
Having good caregiver help is an absolute perk

To process new information a headache for him
Chances for learning anything increasingly slim

Today Jim told the caregiver he does everything wrong
How hard that must be for a man formerly so strong

It is necessary to put directly into his mouth his medication
Even though it may at times cause aggravation

Pills have been dropped on the floor
Our Yorkie snapping them up before

Bringing fright and Vet bills when she eats
To her, no difference between meds and treats

Today, on rifles and guns Jim fixated
Reminding my daughter; safety dictated

Who Am I and where are We Now?

Jim might ask:

Who am I; where are we now?
Everything seems strange somehow

My mind speaks to me—this or that
But not instructions of how to get at

Neither rhyme nor reason the cells to fail
Try with all my might, still can't prevail

Impossible for mere mortals to foresee
The times or impairments to what degree

~*~

I might say:

Been asked many times how long will Jim live?
Seriously? An expiration date the Lord didn't give

"Will he have to go into a facility?" they ask of me
Crystal ball not working, the future I can't foresee

I feel sorry for those not enjoying each day
Regrets they may have some along the way

Now is the time! Don't throw away today
Tomorrow may be too late for a love display

Some quick to critique the care that I give
Only hoping me; he'll still outlive

Narcissistic persons will never understand
Only thought is for inheritance in their hand

~*~

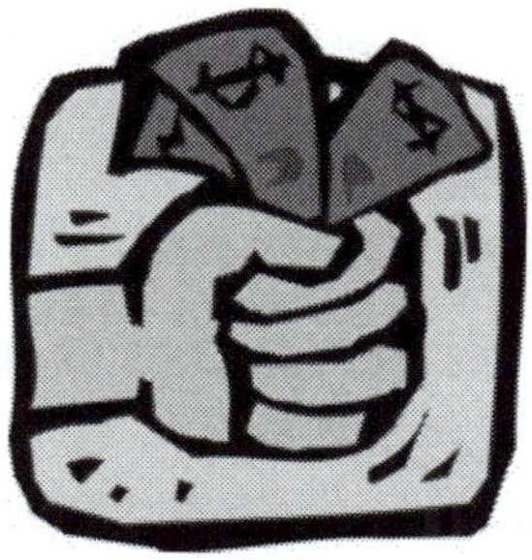

~*~*~*~*~

I Want To Go Home

Multiple times—every day—my loved one
exclaims, "I want to go home"
I explain that we ***are*** home; he doesn't believe
me and wants to roam

With his awful hallucinations and the paranoia it
brings
Home to him is not just a house of familiar things

Home is a *symbolic place* to obtain peace
He hopes then; the awful aberrations will cease

Whenever he is tired or anxious it is worse
That damn Dementia; what a horrendous curse!

Truly it's not a disease affecting an individual
Claiming the caregiver-spouse too; unequivocal

Statistics claim that—40% of caregivers die first
The Alzheimer's patient will not be cognizant of
the worst

God—do you hear me—it hurts! 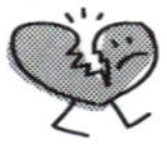

Karen J. Chism 10/27/2014

I Live Alone

The man I fell in love with and married
Has left me alone, although his body has tarried

Each and every day a part of him crumbles
Ever so slowly, to where I know not; he tumbles

He has imaginary friends not introduced to me
I call them *friends* but; to him not friendly, I see

They will anger him often for failing to talk
His descriptions so detailed they often shock

I attempt to engage my love in a conversation
His attempts to communicate cause agitation

He will sit and stare at nothing or what I can't see
Oh God—why all alone did he leave me?

He was my best and *only* friend and lover
I'm like a beacon in the dark as he does hover

He will shadow me so close I turn and he is there
I'm really not alone; he's like the clothes I wear

He is here with me, but yet he is not
Look what that damn Dementia has wrought!

Broken Heart Remedy

My heart was broken; gaping wide
A chasm so deep none could fill
Only the Majesty of Christ should abide

When each new trauma comes into my life
Opening the break; anew
More room for Christ to replace the strife

Turning a seemly bad thing to good
Not understanding at that moment
But God knew that I soon would

Not asking for terrible things to upset my day
Yet with His Grace, His comfort
Everything will turn out okay

Truly—as the Scripture does proclaim
I can do all things, through Christ
Who strengthens me; in Him I'll always remain

Maybe if all seems to be going our way
Our need wouldn't be as obvious
As it is when we have a really bad day

A broken heart can be the worst pain
Speaking of the heart that is connected to the brain
That can be fixed by calling on Jesus' name!

Karen J. Chism 5/12/14

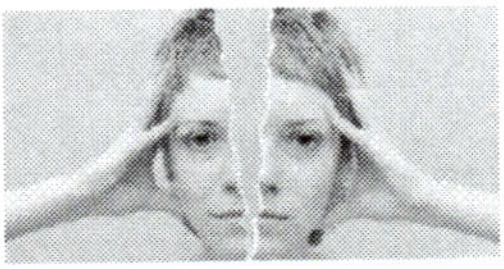

[I know deep in my heart that it is solely because of mine and my husband's abiding faith in Jesus Christ, as our Lord and personal Savior that we are able to withstand the rigors of these horrific diseases that we are both afflicted with. He picks us back up when Dementia and Cancer have knocked us down; He gives us strength and eternal hope. We pray for only His will to be done.]

Thank You

I would like to thank each and every one of you for your interest in my writings. An *honest review* on the site from which you purchased my book, would be greatly appreciated. *Even one line of feedback means so much to me!* May God bless each and every one of you!

Love ya, Karen

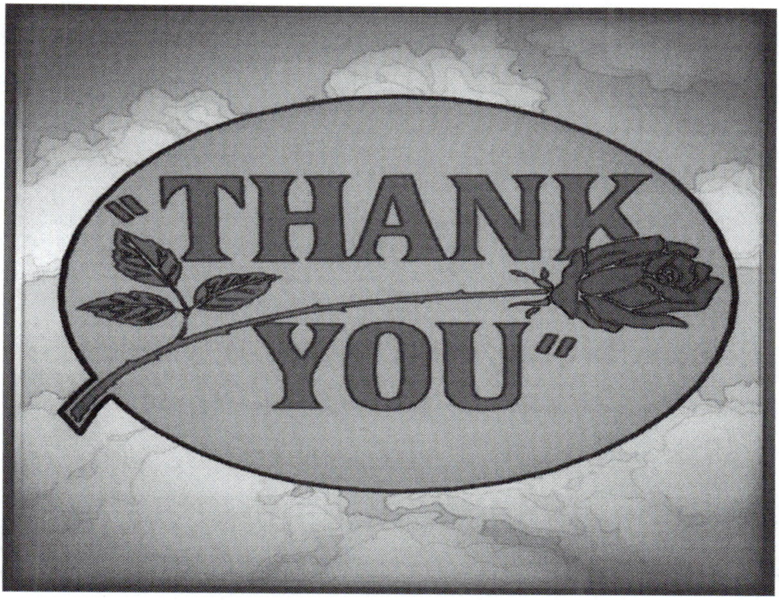

Note From the Editor

This book has been a challenge for me to edit because I am personally connected to the topic of which it speaks. You see, I am Karen's daughter and Jim is my step-father. I love them both with all my heart. My heart is weighed down, with empathy for them; and also a sense of personal loss and grief; because, this disease affects more than just the individual it afflicts.

I am so proud of my Mom for writing this book because I truly believe it will help some people understand Dementia better.

I say this because, while in college I read about many different learning styles; confirming in my mind what I already had observed – not all individuals learn in the same manner. Therefore, one person may be best able to glean an understanding of Dementia by reading a medical textbook, while another may understand best by listening to a song, reading a poem, or taking in a novel/movie such as "Still Alice."[2] Others still, may learn best by observation, or even from personal experience.

I know that someone will be touched by my Mom's writings and will be left with a greater understanding, compassion, and empathy for individuals, their families, and caregivers that are in the grips of the horrible diseases of the mind.

Unfortunately, sometimes even close relatives only have a limited view or understanding of the depths of the devastation these types of diseases can bring. I say this because, even if they visit their loved one on a regular basis, or perhaps even daily for a few hours, one cannot truly comprehend it all unless they live with the person. I have been fortunate enough to be able to travel frequently to stay with Mom and Dad for weeks and months at a time; thus truly witnessing 24/7 how the patient is affected by the disease; also, experiencing first hand, a small degree of caregiver burn-out.

I've heard many medical professionals caution, "There will be many ups and downs with these types of diseases . . . good days and bad days . . ." I can certainly attest to the fact that their predictions were true—every day is a new *adventure.* However; I really was not prepared for the realization *that each and every hour, or even minute, can* — and often does offer startling contrasts; bringing new challenges and obstacles to overcome or adjust to.

Dad is an exceptionally brilliant man and one of my life's great joys has been the deep and interesting talks and debates we have shared over the years. He has taught me much about life, health and wellness; and most importantly about the Holy Bible, and my Christian walk.

Oh, how I miss those times spent conversing; but you see . . . Dad now appears to be a prisoner in his own mind. Occasionally, the Dementia will grant him a *day pass*, so to speak, and for a few moments, we are able to share a brief, but cherished conversation . . . then, the next moment he'll have forgotten what we had just discussed! As the days and his disease progresses, these short glimpses of his true self become much more elusive.

How excruciating it must be for Dad to live inside his demented mind, with the confusion, anxiety, and frustration of not being able to communicate effectively; or even be able to trust his perceptions of the world around him. All the while, realizing (still as of this writing) the awful fate that awaits him.

He said to me the other day, *[while holding his hand up to gesture an inch]* "When there is the slightest external stress, commotion, or controversy — it creates a huge stress in my brain" *[gesturing again, a six inch space between his thumb and forefinger].* Later that day he expressed, "It's awful this thing! *[Dementia]* I can feel it taking hold and gaining ground!"

How shocking it always is for me to see how much further the disease has progressed, and how much less of Dad I recognize, from one visit to the next. I brace myself for the day when he no longer smiles in acknowledgement when I walk into the room. I know eventually he will not know who I am; that is why each time I hear him say, "I love you honey," I know how fortunate I still am.

In the short time it has taken to finish preparing this book for publication many changes have taken place. Now Dad and I can only share a few words at best. He needs assistance with all of his activities of daily living. Taking him to the park for a walk is now quite a gamble—down the walk to the driveway is about all we can handle. It is hard to gain or keep his attention, and he has difficulty expressing his needs. I sometimes feel helpless, not being able to make life better for him. I cannot even imagine what he is feeling.

Then there's my Mom who endures watching her husband leaving her in bits and pieces to never return. Yet, she is ever patient, loving, and kind in her caring for Dad; even at the expense of her own health. Being his caregiver without a doubt has hastened the progression of her disease. Such a loving example of true sacrificial love!

Life is so hard for the spouse because they become a victim, by way of the *collateral-damage* the disease leaves in its wake. Being a caregiver is hard, but what people don't realize is that the "*war-weary*" spouse is the <u>primary</u> caregiver and the job is 24/7! Gone are the days when at the end of the day, she can unwind and share with her spouse the job woes or stresses of the day; because he isn't be able to comprehend.

It's as if this disease holds everyone it touches in a perpetual state of grief; not allowing them to move through the different stages. *I equate it to going to a funeral every day.* This is most unhealthy and almost too much to bare.

As I watch my parents struggle with Cancer and Dementia, I can say that Dementia is by far the cruelest thing I've ever seen. Quite honestly, if it weren't for my faith in Christ, I don't know how I would survive.

God is faithful and good!

K. Compton –
Editor in Chief, Heartspeak Publications Incorporated

Helpful Resources on Dementia, Alzheimer's, and Aging

Alzheimer's Association
www.alz.org

Alzheimer's Foundation of America
www.alzfdn.org

Alzheimer's & Dementia Journal
www.alzheimersanddementia.com

Bright Focus Foundation
www.brightfocus.org

Centers for Disease Control and Prevention
www.cdc.gov

Facebook Alzheimer's Awareness Community
www.facebook.com/fightalzheimers

Lewy Body Dementia Association, Inc.
www.lbda.org

National Caregivers Library
www.caregiverslibrary.org

National Institutes of Health - Clinical Center

www.cc.nih.gov

National Institute on Aging

www.nia.nih.gov

NIH Senior Health

www.nihseniorhealth.gov

National Institute of Neurological Disorders and Stroke

www.ninds.nih.gov

National Council on Aging

http://www.ncoa.org

Teepa Snow (care expert)

www.teepasnow.com

U.S. Department of Veterans Affairs Caregiver Support Services

http://www.caregiver.va.gov/support/support_services.asp

Author's Bibliography

Other Large Print books by Karen J. Chism:

Nonfiction Poetry

Reflections In My Twilight Years-collection One
Reflections In My Twilight Years-collection Two
Reflections In My Twilight Years-collection Three

> (All three collections of the Reflections series are also available in a single volume e-book)

The Rhythm of Life

A Memoir

Is She Dead Yet, When The Children Want Your Money Before You Die

You are invited to visit my website www.karenchism.com for updates and my blog.

Publisher Information

If you would like to receive updates concerning future offerings by Heartspeak Publications Incorporated or this author; ask to be added to our mailing list by sending an e-mail to:
heartspeakpublications@gmail.com

Heartspeak Publications Incorporated
Logo design by: K. Compton

References

[1] **"I'm Not Gonna Miss You"** Songwriters: Raymond, Julian / Campbell, Glen - Published by: Lyrics © Warner/Chappell Music, Inc.

"I'm Not Gonna Miss You"

I'm still here, but yet I'm gone
I don't play guitar or sing my songs
They never defined who I am
The man that loves you 'til the end

You're the last person I will love
You're the last face I will recall
And best of all, I'm not gonna miss you
Not gonna miss you

I'm never gonna hold you like I did
Or say I love you to the kids
You're never gonna see it in my eyes
It's not gonna hurt me when you cry

I'm never gonna know what you go through
All the things I say or do
All the hurt and all the pain
One thing selfishly remains

I'm not gonna miss you
I'm not gonna miss you

Source: MetroLyrics.com

[2] "Still Alice" By Lisa Genova

[3] "Window of Opportunity: Living with the reality of Parkinson's and the threat of dementia" By Kirk Hall

This is not the final chapter to this damn Dementia story
Whatever events unfold—we can look forward to Glory!

Made in the USA
Monee, IL
04 November 2026

67386061R10042